THIS PLANNER

Belongs To:

I'm PREGNANT!

HOW I FOUND OUT

MY REACTION

DUE DATE

WHAT I AM MOST EXCITED ABOUT

WHO I TOLD FIRST

WHAT I WANT YOU BOTH TO KNOW

MY BIRTH PLAN Ideas

WHO I WANT IN THE DELIVERY ROOM:

TYPE OF BIRTH

- ☐ VAGINAL
- ☐ WATER BIRTH
- ☐ C-SECTION
- ☐ VBAC

THOUGHTS ABOUT BIRTH AND WHAT IS MOST IMPORTANT TO ME

GETTING READY FOR THE BIG DAY: TO DO

NOTES & IDEAS (lighting, music, etc.)

PREGNANCY Tracker

40 Weeks

Keep track of how you're feeling every week of your pregnancy.

APPOINTMENT Tracker

Keep track of your pre-natal classes and doctor appointments.

DATE	TIME	ADDRESS	PURPOSE

BABY SHOPPING *List*

Start planning for the arrival of your baby by using the shopping list below.

☐ Undershirts	☐ Crib	☐ Bottles
☐ Socks	☐ Bassinet	☐ Bottle Liners
☐ Pajamas	☐ Baby Bath tub	☐ Nursing Bra & Pads
☐ Sweaters	☐ Car Seat	☐ Breast Pump
☐ Onesies	☐ Stroller	☐ Formula
☐ Hats	☐ High Chair	☐ Pacifiers
☐ Bibs	☐ Play Pen	☐ Bottle Brush
☐ Blanket	☐ Baby Swing	☐ Burp Cloths
☐ Diaper Bag	☐ Monitor	☐ Bottle Sanitizer
☐ Mitts	☐ Change Table	☐ Nipples
☐ Diapers	☐ Rocking Chair	☐ Baby Powder
☐ Booties	☐ Night Light	☐ Baby Wipes
☐ Receiving Blankets	☐ Mobile	
☐ Crib Sheet	☐ Bouncer	
☐ Wash Cloths	☐ Nail Clippers	
☐ Towels	☐ Teething Toys	
	☐ Baby Wipes	
	☐ Diaper Pail	

Weight PREGNANCY Tracker

Weight Tracker Chart

It's important to keep track of your weight throughout your pregnancy. Record your weight in the chart below every week, starting at week 4.

WEEKLY WEIGHT TRACKER

Week		Week		Week		Week		Week	
4		12		20		28		36	
5		13		21		29		37	
6		14		22		30		38	
7		15		23		31		39	
8		16		24		32		40	
9		17		25		33			
10		18		26		34			
11		19		27		35			

NOTE: According to the American Pregnancy Association, pregnant women should consume up to 300 more calories a day. Further, healthy eating is critical to your baby's development which means you should make sure to maintain a well-balanced diet, high in nutrients and proteins.

HEALTHY FOOD Ideas

VEGETABLES & LOW SUGAR FRUIT	PROTEINS	COMPLEX CARBS	HEALTHY FATS	SUPPLEMENTS
Leafy greens (spinach, etc.)	Organic meat	Beets	Avocado	Vitamin D
Broccoli	Liver	Carrots	Olive Oil	Fish Oil
Cauliflower	Bone Broth	Sweet Potatoes	Coconut Oil	Algae Oil
Cabbage	Beans	Yams	Yogurt	Probiotics
Asparagus	Lentils	Parsnips	Almonds	Ginger Pills
Cucumber	Flax Seed	Turnips	Mixed Nuts	Licorice Root
Mushrooms	Pumpkin Seed	Pumpkin	Soybean	Magnesium
Celery	Chia Seed	Buckwheat	Olives	Krill Oil
Radish	Salmon	Brown Rice	Nut butter	Iron Pills
Grapefruit & Melon	Herring	Squash		
Berries (all kinds)				
Peaches (with skin)				

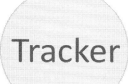

Tracker | PRE-NATAL *Visits*

♥♥♥♥♥ *Important Dates* ♥♥♥♥♥

Keep track of your pre-natal appointments and include a summary of each visit.

DATE		SUMMARY OF APPOINTMENT
HOW FAR ALONG?		
YOUR WEIGHT		
BLOOD PRESSURE		
FETAL HEART RATE		
DOCTOR		

NOTES:

NEXT APPOINTMENT.:

DATE		SUMMARY OF APPOINTMENT
HOW FAR ALONG?		
YOUR WEIGHT		
BLOOD PRESSURE		
FETAL HEART RATE		
DOCTOR		

NOTES:

NEXT APPOINTMENT.:

DATE		SUMMARY OF APPOINTMENT
HOW FAR ALONG?		
YOUR WEIGHT		
BLOOD PRESSURE		
FETAL HEART RATE		
DOCTOR		

NOTES:

NEXT APPOINTMENT.:

FIRST *Trimester*

1-13 Weeks

Journal your thoughts and feelings during each trimester so you can later reflect on your pregnancy journey.

HOW I FELT DURING MY FIRST TRIMESTER

MY FAVORITE MEMORIES

SYMPTOMS & CRAVINGS

ENERGY
♥ ♥ ♥ ♥ ♥ ♥

SLEEP
♥ ♥ ♥ ♥ ♥ ♥

CRAVINGS
♥ ♥ ♥ ♥ ♥ ♥

MOODS
♥ ♥ ♥ ♥ ♥ ♥

TO DO LIST: 1st TRIMESTER

FIRST TRIMESTER *Photos*

MEMORIES ARE FOREVER

SECOND *Trimester*

14-27 Weeks

HOW I FELT DURING MY SECOND TRIMESTER

MY FAVORITE MEMORIES

SYMPTOMS & CRAVINGS

ENERGY
♥ ♥ ♥ ♥ ♥ ♥

SLEEP
♥ ♥ ♥ ♥ ♥ ♥

CRAVINGS
♥ ♥ ♥ ♥ ♥ ♥

MOODS
♥ ♥ ♥ ♥ ♥ ♥

TO DO LIST: 2nd TRIMESTER

SECOND TRIMESTER *Photos*

MEMORIES ARE FOREVER

28-40 Weeks

THIRD Trimester

HOW I FELT DURING MY THIRD TRIMESTER

MY FAVORITE MEMORIES

SYMPTOMS & CRAVINGS

ENERGY

SLEEP

CRAVINGS

MOODS

TO DO LIST: 3rd TRIMESTER

THIRD TRIMESTER *Photos*

MEMORIES ARE FOREVER

MY BABY Shower

BABY SHOWER PHOTOS

GAMES PLAYED

ON THE MENU

HIGHLIGHTS & MEMORIES

MY BABY Shower Gifts

Keep track of your baby shower gifts and send thank you notes

NAME	GIFT	ADDRESS	SENT?
			☐
			☐
			☐
			☐
			☐
			☐
			☐
			☐
			☐
			☐
			☐
			☐
			☐
			☐

NURSERY *Planner*

COLOR SCHEME IDEAS:

ITEM TO PURCHASE	PRICE	NOTES

FURNITURE IDEAS

DECORATIVE IDEAS

BABY NAME Ideas

TOP 3 BOY NAMES			
	NAME MEANINGS		

TOP 3 GIRL NAMES			
	NAME MEANINGS		

BABY NAME RESOURCES (LIST YOUR FAVORITE PARENTING & PREGNANCY WEBSITES):

OTHER BOY NAME POSSIBILITIES	OTHER GIRL NAME POSSIBILITES

HOSPITAL *Checklist*

FOR ME	FOR PARTNER	FOR BABIES

PREGNANCY SHOPPING *List*

BABY CLOTHING	SUPPLIES/MEDICATION	FURNITURE/TOYS

FIRST TRIMESTER SHOPPING	SECOND TRIMESTER SHOPPING	THIRD TRIMESTER SHOPPING

Tracker | FETAL *Movement*

Starting around week 16, keep track of when you feel your baby move.

WEEK 16	TIME	NOTES
MON		
TUE		
WED		
THU		
FRI		
SAT		
SUN		

WEEK 17	TIME	NOTES
MON		
TUE		
WED		
THU		
FRI		
SAT		
SUN		

WEEK 18	TIME	NOTES
MON		
TUE		
WED		
THU		
FRI		
SAT		
SUN		

WEEK 19	TIME	NOTES
MON		
TUE		
WED		
THU		
FRI		
SAT		
SUN		

WEEK 20	TIME	NOTES
MON		
TUE		
WED		
THU		
FRI		
SAT		
SUN		

WEEK 21	TIME	NOTES
MON		
TUE		
WED		
THU		
FRI		
SAT		
SUN		

WEEK 22	TIME	NOTES
MON		
TUE		
WED		
THU		
FRI		
SAT		
SUN		

WEEK 23	TIME	NOTES
MON		
TUE		
WED		
THU		
FRI		
SAT		
SUN		

WEEK 24	TIME	NOTES
MON		
TUE		
WED		
THU		
FRI		
SAT		
SUN		

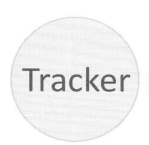

FETAL Movement
Tracker

WEEK 25	TIME	NOTES
MON		
TUE		
WED		
THU		
FRI		
SAT		
SUN		

WEEK 26	TIME	NOTES
MON		
TUE		
WED		
THU		
FRI		
SAT		
SUN		

WEEK 27	TIME	NOTES
MON		
TUE		
WED		
THU		
FRI		
SAT		
SUN		

WEEK 28	TIME	NOTES
MON		
TUE		
WED		
THU		
FRI		
SAT		
SUN		

WEEK 29	TIME	NOTES
MON		
TUE		
WED		
THU		
FRI		
SAT		
SUN		

WEEK 30	TIME	NOTES
MON		
TUE		
WED		
THU		
FRI		
SAT		
SUN		

WEEK 31	TIME	NOTES
MON		
TUE		
WED		
THU		
FRI		
SAT		
SUN		

WEEK 32	TIME	NOTES
MON		
TUE		
WED		
THU		
FRI		
SAT		
SUN		

WEEK 33	TIME	NOTES
MON		
TUE		
WED		
THU		
FRI		
SAT		
SUN		

Tracker : FETAL Movement

WEEK 34	TIME	NOTES
MON		
TUE		
WED		
THU		
FRI		
SAT		
SUN		

WEEK 35	TIME	NOTES
MON		
TUE		
WED		
THU		
FRI		
SAT		
SUN		

WEEK 36	TIME	NOTES
MON		
TUE		
WED		
THU		
FRI		
SAT		
SUN		

WEEK 37	TIME	NOTES
MON		
TUE		
WED		
THU		
FRI		
SAT		
SUN		

WEEK 38	TIME	NOTES
MON		
TUE		
WED		
THU		
FRI		
SAT		
SUN		

WEEK 39	TIME	NOTES
MON		
TUE		
WED		
THU		
FRI		
SAT		
SUN		

WEEK 40	TIME	NOTES
MON		
TUE		
WED		
THU		
FRI		
SAT		
SUN		

NOTES

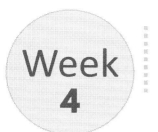

PREGNANCY *Journal*

Week 4

TOTAL WEIGHT GAIN

BELLY MEASUREMENT

BABY BUMP PHOTO

WEEKLY REFLECTIONS

SYMPTOMS & CRAVINGS

WHAT I WANT TO REMEMBER MOST

I'M MOST EXCITED ABOUT

I'M MOST NERVOUS ABOUT

Dear Babies,

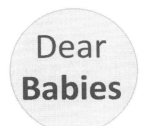

PREGNANCY *Journal*

TODAY'S DATE

WEEKS PREGNANT

HOW I'M FEELING TODAY

What I want you both to know

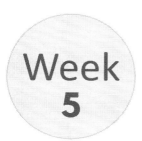

PREGNANCY *Journal*

Week 5

TOTAL WEIGHT GAIN

BELLY MEASUREMENT

BABY BUMP PHOTO

WEEKLY REFLECTIONS

SYMPTOMS & CRAVINGS

WHAT I WANT TO REMEMBER MOST

I'M MOST EXCITED ABOUT

I'M MOST NERVOUS ABOUT

Dear Babies,

Dear Babies

PREGNANCY *Journal*

TODAY'S DATE

WEEKS PREGNANT

HOW I'M FEELING TODAY

What I want you both to know

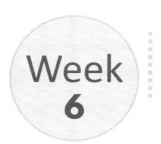

PREGNANCY *Journal*

Week 6

TOTAL WEIGHT GAIN

BELLY MEASUREMENT

BABY BUMP PHOTO

WEEKLY REFLECTIONS

SYMPTOMS & CRAVINGS

WHAT I WANT TO REMEMBER MOST

I'M MOST EXCITED ABOUT

I'M MOST NERVOUS ABOUT

Dear Babies,

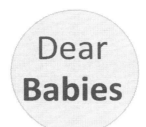

PREGNANCY *Journal*

TODAY'S DATE

WEEKS PREGNANT

HOW I'M FEELING TODAY

What I want you both to know

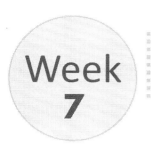

PREGNANCY Journal

Week 7

TOTAL WEIGHT GAIN

BELLY MEASUREMENT

BABY BUMP PHOTO

WEEKLY REFLECTIONS

SYMPTOMS & CRAVINGS

WHAT I WANT TO REMEMBER MOST

I'M MOST EXCITED ABOUT

I'M MOST NERVOUS ABOUT

Dear Babies,

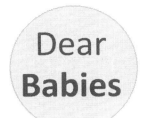

PREGNANCY *Journal*

TODAY'S DATE

WEEKS PREGNANT

HOW I'M FEELING TODAY

What I want you both to know

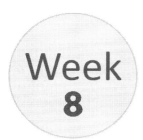

Week 8

PREGNANCY *Journal*

TOTAL WEIGHT GAIN

BELLY MEASUREMENT

BABY BUMP PHOTO

WEEKLY REFLECTIONS

SYMPTOMS & CRAVINGS

WHAT I WANT TO REMEMBER MOST

I'M MOST EXCITED ABOUT

I'M MOST NERVOUS ABOUT

Dear Babies,

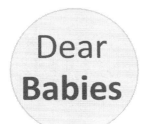

PREGNANCY *Journal*

TODAY'S DATE

WEEKS PREGNANT

HOW I'M FEELING TODAY

What I want you both to know

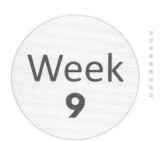

PREGNANCY *Journal*

Week 9

TOTAL WEIGHT GAIN

BELLY MEASUREMENT

BABY BUMP PHOTO

WEEKLY REFLECTIONS

SYMPTOMS & CRAVINGS

WHAT I WANT TO REMEMBER MOST

I'M MOST EXCITED ABOUT

I'M MOST NERVOUS ABOUT

Dear Babies,

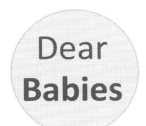

PREGNANCY *Journal*

TODAY'S DATE

WEEKS PREGNANT

HOW I'M FEELING TODAY

What I want you both to know

Week 10 | PREGNANCY *Journal*

TOTAL WEIGHT GAIN

BELLY MEASUREMENT

BABY BUMP PHOTO

WEEKLY REFLECTIONS

SYMPTOMS & CRAVINGS

WHAT I WANT TO REMEMBER MOST

I'M MOST EXCITED ABOUT

I'M MOST NERVOUS ABOUT

Dear Babies,

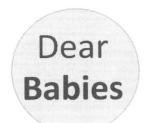

PREGNANCY *Journal*

TODAY'S DATE

WEEKS PREGNANT

HOW I'M FEELING TODAY

What I want you both to know

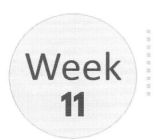

PREGNANCY *Journal*

Week 11

TOTAL WEIGHT GAIN

BELLY MEASUREMENT

BABY BUMP PHOTO

WEEKLY REFLECTIONS

SYMPTOMS & CRAVINGS

WHAT I WANT TO REMEMBER MOST

I'M MOST EXCITED ABOUT

I'M MOST NERVOUS ABOUT

Dear Babies

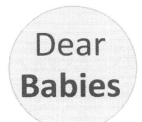

PREGNANCY *Journal*

TODAY'S DATE

WEEKS PREGNANT

HOW I'M FEELING TODAY

What I want you both to know

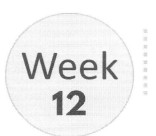

PREGNANCY *Journal*

Week 12

TOTAL WEIGHT GAIN

BELLY MEASUREMENT

BABY BUMP PHOTO

WEEKLY REFLECTIONS

SYMPTOMS & CRAVINGS

WHAT I WANT TO REMEMBER MOST

I'M MOST EXCITED ABOUT

I'M MOST NERVOUS ABOUT

Dear Babies,

12 WEEKS | ULTRASOUND *Scan*

ULTRASOUND PHOTO

ULTRASOUND RESULTS

BABY A's LENGTH: B:

BABY A'S WEIGHT: B:

BPD:

DUE DATE:

Notes

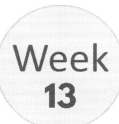

Week 13 | PREGNANCY *Journal*

TOTAL WEIGHT GAIN

BELLY MEASUREMENT

BABY BUMP PHOTO

WEEKLY REFLECTIONS

SYMPTOMS & CRAVINGS

WHAT I WANT TO REMEMBER MOST

I'M MOST EXCITED ABOUT

I'M MOST NERVOUS ABOUT

Dear Babies

Dear Babies

PREGNANCY *Journal*

TODAY'S DATE

WEEKS PREGNANT

HOW I'M FEELING TODAY

What I want you both to know

Week 14 | PREGNANCY *Journal*

TOTAL WEIGHT GAIN

BELLY MEASUREMENT

BABY BUMP PHOTO

WEEKLY REFLECTIONS

SYMPTOMS & CRAVINGS

WHAT I WANT TO REMEMBER MOST

I'M MOST EXCITED ABOUT

I'M MOST NERVOUS ABOUT

Dear Babies,

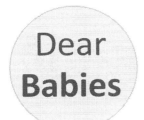

PREGNANCY *Journal*

TODAY'S DATE

WEEKS PREGNANT

HOW I'M FEELING TODAY

What I want you both to know

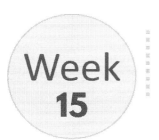

PREGNANCY Journal

Week 15

TOTAL WEIGHT GAIN

BELLY MEASUREMENT

BABY BUMP PHOTO

WEEKLY REFLECTIONS

SYMPTOMS & CRAVINGS

WHAT I WANT TO REMEMBER MOST

I'M MOST EXCITED ABOUT

I'M MOST NERVOUS ABOUT

Dear Babies,

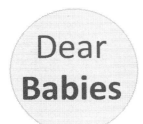

PREGNANCY *Journal*

TODAY'S DATE

WEEKS PREGNANT

HOW I'M FEELING TODAY

What I want you both to know

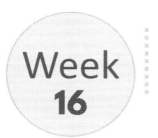

PREGNANCY *Journal*

Week 16

TOTAL WEIGHT GAIN

BELLY MEASUREMENT

BABY BUMP PHOTO

WEEKLY REFLECTIONS

SYMPTOMS & CRAVINGS

WHAT I WANT TO REMEMBER MOST

I'M MOST EXCITED ABOUT

I'M MOST NERVOUS ABOUT

Dear Babies,

Dear Babies

PREGNANCY *Journal*

TODAY'S DATE

WEEKS PREGNANT

HOW I'M FEELING TODAY

What I want you both to know

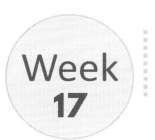

PREGNANCY *Journal*

Week 17

TOTAL WEIGHT GAIN

BELLY MEASUREMENT

BABY BUMP PHOTO

WEEKLY REFLECTIONS

SYMPTOMS & CRAVINGS

WHAT I WANT TO REMEMBER MOST

I'M MOST EXCITED ABOUT

I'M MOST NERVOUS ABOUT

Dear Babies,

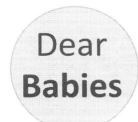

PREGNANCY *Journal*

TODAY'S DATE

WEEKS PREGNANT

HOW I'M FEELING TODAY

What I want you both to know

Week 18 — PREGNANCY *Journal*

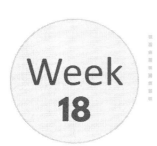

TOTAL WEIGHT GAIN

BELLY MEASUREMENT

BABY BUMP PHOTO

WEEKLY REFLECTIONS

SYMPTOMS & CRAVINGS

WHAT I WANT TO REMEMBER MOST

I'M MOST EXCITED ABOUT

I'M MOST NERVOUS ABOUT

Dear Babies,

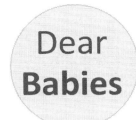

PREGNANCY *Journal*

TODAY'S DATE

WEEKS PREGNANT

HOW I'M FEELING TODAY

What I want you both to know

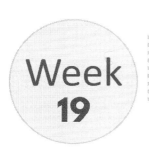

Week 19

PREGNANCY *Journal*

TOTAL WEIGHT GAIN

BELLY MEASUREMENT

BABY BUMP PHOTO

WEEKLY REFLECTIONS

SYMPTOMS & CRAVINGS

WHAT I WANT TO REMEMBER MOST

I'M MOST EXCITED ABOUT

I'M MOST NERVOUS ABOUT

Dear Babies,

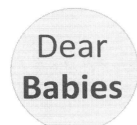

PREGNANCY *Journal*

TODAY'S DATE

WEEKS PREGNANT

HOW I'M FEELING TODAY

What I want you both to know

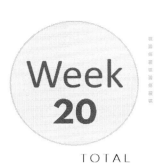

PREGNANCY *Journal*

Week 20

TOTAL WEIGHT GAIN

BELLY MEASUREMENT

BABY BUMP PHOTO

WEEKLY REFLECTIONS

SYMPTOMS & CRAVINGS

WHAT I WANT TO REMEMBER MOST

I'M MOST EXCITED ABOUT

I'M MOST NERVOUS ABOUT

Dear Babies,

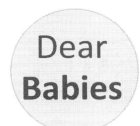

PREGNANCY *Journal*

TODAY'S DATE

WEEKS PREGNANT

HOW I'M FEELING TODAY

What I want you both to know

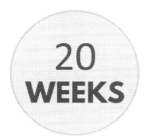

ULTRASOUND Scan

20 WEEKS

ULTRASOUND PHOTO

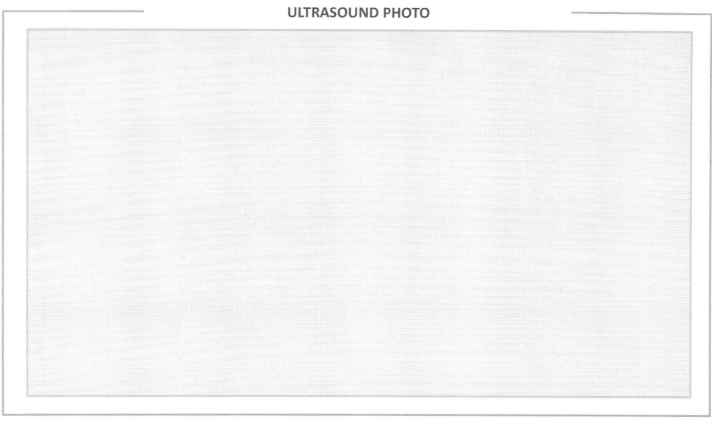

ULTRASOUND RESULTS

BABY A's LENGTH: B:

BABY A's WEIGHT: B:

BPD:

DUE DATE:

Notes

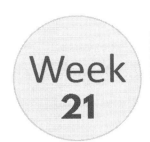

PREGNANCY *Journal*

TOTAL WEIGHT GAIN

BELLY MEASUREMENT

BABY BUMP PHOTO

WEEKLY REFLECTIONS

SYMPTOMS & CRAVINGS

WHAT I WANT TO REMEMBER MOST

Dear Babies,

I'M MOST EXCITED ABOUT

I'M MOST NERVOUS ABOUT

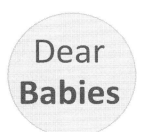

PREGNANCY *Journal*

TODAY'S DATE

WEEKS PREGNANT

HOW I'M FEELING TODAY

What I want you both to know

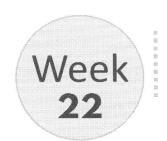

PREGNANCY *Journal*

Week 22

TOTAL WEIGHT GAIN

BELLY MEASUREMENT

BABY BUMP PHOTO

WEEKLY REFLECTIONS

SYMPTOMS & CRAVINGS

WHAT I WANT TO REMEMBER MOST

I'M MOST EXCITED ABOUT

I'M MOST NERVOUS ABOUT

Dear Babies

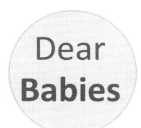

PREGNANCY *Journal*

TODAY'S DATE

WEEKS PREGNANT

HOW I'M FEELING TODAY

What I want you both to know

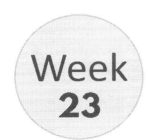

PREGNANCY *Journal*

Week 23

TOTAL WEIGHT GAIN

BELLY MEASUREMENT

BABY BUMP PHOTO

WEEKLY REFLECTIONS

SYMPTOMS & CRAVINGS

WHAT I WANT TO REMEMBER MOST

I'M MOST EXCITED ABOUT

I'M MOST NERVOUS ABOUT

Dear Babies,

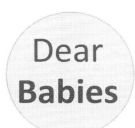

PREGNANCY *Journal*

TODAY'S DATE

WEEKS PREGNANT

HOW I'M FEELING TODAY

What I want you both to know

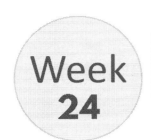

PREGNANCY *Journal*

Week 24

TOTAL WEIGHT GAIN

BELLY MEASUREMENT

BABY BUMP PHOTO

WEEKLY REFLECTIONS

SYMPTOMS & CRAVINGS

WHAT I WANT TO REMEMBER MOST

I'M MOST EXCITED ABOUT

I'M MOST NERVOUS ABOUT

Dear Babies,

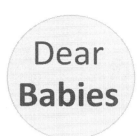

PREGNANCY *Journal*

TODAY'S DATE

WEEKS PREGNANT

HOW I'M FEELING TODAY

What I want you both to know

Week 25 — PREGNANCY *Journal*

TOTAL WEIGHT GAIN

BELLY MEASUREMENT

BABY BUMP PHOTO

WEEKLY REFLECTIONS

SYMPTOMS & CRAVINGS

WHAT I WANT TO REMEMBER MOST

I'M MOST EXCITED ABOUT

I'M MOST NERVOUS ABOUT

Dear Babies,

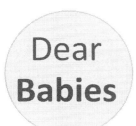

PREGNANCY *Journal*

Dear Babies

TODAY'S DATE

WEEKS PREGNANT

HOW I'M FEELING TODAY

What I want you both to know

Week 26 — PREGNANCY *Journal*

TOTAL WEIGHT GAIN

BELLY MEASUREMENT

BABY BUMP PHOTO

WEEKLY REFLECTIONS

SYMPTOMS & CRAVINGS

WHAT I WANT TO REMEMBER MOST

I'M MOST EXCITED ABOUT

I'M MOST NERVOUS ABOUT

Dear Babies,

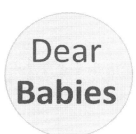

PREGNANCY *Journal*

TODAY'S DATE

WEEKS PREGNANT

HOW I'M FEELING TODAY

What I want you both to know

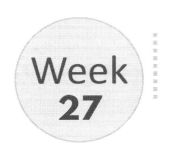

PREGNANCY *Journal*

Week 27

TOTAL WEIGHT GAIN

BELLY MEASUREMENT

BABY BUMP PHOTO

WEEKLY REFLECTIONS

SYMPTOMS & CRAVINGS

WHAT I WANT TO REMEMBER MOST

I'M MOST EXCITED ABOUT

I'M MOST NERVOUS ABOUT

Dear Babies,

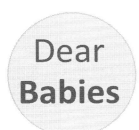

PREGNANCY *Journal*

TODAY'S DATE

WEEKS PREGNANT

HOW I'M FEELING TODAY

What I want you both to know

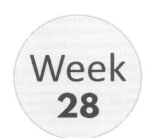

PREGNANCY Journal

Week 28

TOTAL WEIGHT GAIN

BELLY MEASUREMENT

BABY BUMP PHOTO

WEEKLY REFLECTIONS

SYMPTOMS & CRAVINGS

WHAT I WANT TO REMEMBER MOST

I'M MOST EXCITED ABOUT

I'M MOST NERVOUS ABOUT

Dear Babies,

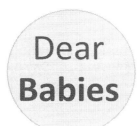

PREGNANCY *Journal*

TODAY'S DATE

WEEKS PREGNANT

HOW I'M FEELING TODAY

What I want you both to know

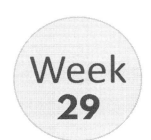

PREGNANCY *Journal*

Week 29

TOTAL WEIGHT GAIN

BELLY MEASUREMENT

BABY BUMP PHOTO

WEEKLY REFLECTIONS

SYMPTOMS & CRAVINGS

WHAT I WANT TO REMEMBER MOST

I'M MOST EXCITED ABOUT

I'M MOST NERVOUS ABOUT

Dear Babies,

Dear Babies
PREGNANCY *Journal*

TODAY'S DATE	WEEKS PREGNANT	HOW I'M FEELING TODAY

What I want you both to know

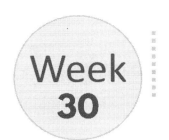

PREGNANCY *Journal*

Week 30

TOTAL WEIGHT GAIN

BELLY MEASUREMENT

BABY BUMP PHOTO

WEEKLY REFLECTIONS

SYMPTOMS & CRAVINGS

WHAT I WANT TO REMEMBER MOST

I'M MOST EXCITED ABOUT

I'M MOST NERVOUS ABOUT

Dear Babies,

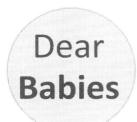

PREGNANCY *Journal*

TODAY'S DATE

WEEKS PREGNANT

HOW I'M FEELING TODAY

What I want you both to know

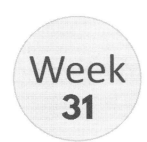

PREGNANCY *Journal*

Week 31

TOTAL WEIGHT GAIN

BELLY MEASUREMENT

BABY BUMP PHOTO

WEEKLY REFLECTIONS

SYMPTOMS & CRAVINGS

WHAT I WANT TO REMEMBER MOST

I'M MOST EXCITED ABOUT

I'M MOST NERVOUS ABOUT

Dear Babies,

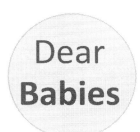

PREGNANCY *Journal*

TODAY'S DATE

WEEKS PREGNANT

HOW I'M FEELING TODAY

What I want you both to know

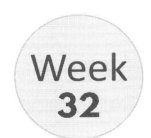

PREGNANCY *Journal*

Week 32

TOTAL WEIGHT GAIN

BELLY MEASUREMENT

BABY BUMP PHOTO

WEEKLY REFLECTIONS

SYMPTOMS & CRAVINGS

WHAT I WANT TO REMEMBER MOST

I'M MOST EXCITED ABOUT

I'M MOST NERVOUS ABOUT

Dear Babies

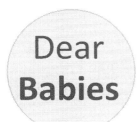

PREGNANCY *Journal*

TODAY'S DATE

WEEKS PREGNANT

HOW I'M FEELING TODAY

What I want you both to know

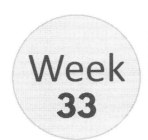

PREGNANCY *Journal*

Week 33

TOTAL WEIGHT GAIN

BELLY MEASUREMENT

BABY BUMP PHOTO

WEEKLY REFLECTIONS

SYMPTOMS & CRAVINGS

WHAT I WANT TO REMEMBER MOST

I'M MOST EXCITED ABOUT

I'M MOST NERVOUS ABOUT

Dear Babies,

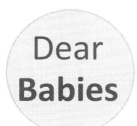

PREGNANCY *Journal*

TODAY'S DATE

WEEKS PREGNANT

HOW I'M FEELING TODAY

What I want you both to know

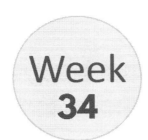

PREGNANCY *Journal*

Week 34

TOTAL WEIGHT GAIN

BELLY MEASUREMENT

BABY BUMP PHOTO

WEEKLY REFLECTIONS

SYMPTOMS & CRAVINGS

WHAT I WANT TO REMEMBER MOST

I'M MOST EXCITED ABOUT

I'M MOST NERVOUS ABOUT

Dear Babies,

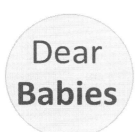

PREGNANCY *Journal*

TODAY'S DATE

WEEKS PREGNANT

HOW I'M FEELING TODAY

What I want you both to know

PREGNANCY *Journal*

Week 35

TOTAL WEIGHT GAIN

BELLY MEASUREMENT

BABY BUMP PHOTO

WEEKLY REFLECTIONS

SYMPTOMS & CRAVINGS

WHAT I WANT TO REMEMBER MOST

I'M MOST EXCITED ABOUT

I'M MOST NERVOUS ABOUT

Dear Babies,

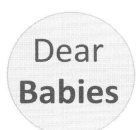

PREGNANCY *Journal*

TODAY'S DATE

WEEKS PREGNANT

HOW I'M FEELING TODAY

What I want you both to know

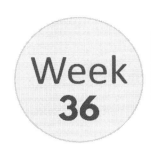

PREGNANCY *Journal*

Week 36

TOTAL WEIGHT GAIN

BELLY MEASUREMENT

BABY BUMP PHOTO

WEEKLY REFLECTIONS

SYMPTOMS & CRAVINGS

WHAT I WANT TO REMEMBER MOST

I'M MOST EXCITED ABOUT

I'M MOST NERVOUS ABOUT

Dear Babies,

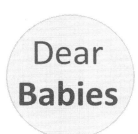

PREGNANCY *Journal*

TODAY'S DATE

WEEKS PREGNANT

HOW I'M FEELING TODAY

What I want you both to know

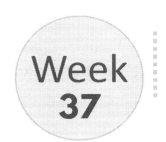

PREGNANCY *Journal*

Week 37

TOTAL WEIGHT GAIN

BELLY MEASUREMENT

BABY BUMP PHOTO

WEEKLY REFLECTIONS

SYMPTOMS & CRAVINGS

WHAT I WANT TO REMEMBER MOST

I'M MOST EXCITED ABOUT

I'M MOST NERVOUS ABOUT

Dear Babies,

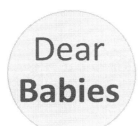

PREGNANCY *Journal*

TODAY'S DATE

WEEKS PREGNANT

HOW I'M FEELING TODAY

What I want you both to know

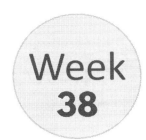

Week 38 — PREGNANCY *Journal*

TOTAL WEIGHT GAIN

BELLY MEASUREMENT

BABY BUMP PHOTO

WEEKLY REFLECTIONS

SYMPTOMS & CRAVINGS

WHAT I WANT TO REMEMBER MOST

I'M MOST EXCITED ABOUT

I'M MOST NERVOUS ABOUT

Dear Babies,

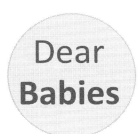

PREGNANCY *Journal*

TODAY'S DATE

WEEKS PREGNANT

HOW I'M FEELING TODAY

What I want you both to know

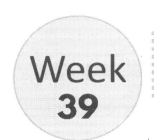

PREGNANCY *Journal*

Week 39

TOTAL WEIGHT GAIN

BELLY MEASUREMENT

BABY BUMP PHOTO

WEEKLY REFLECTIONS

SYMPTOMS & CRAVINGS

WHAT I WANT TO REMEMBER MOST

I'M MOST EXCITED ABOUT

I'M MOST NERVOUS ABOUT

Dear Babies,

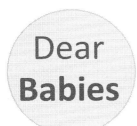

PREGNANCY *Journal*

TODAY'S DATE

WEEKS PREGNANT

HOW I'M FEELING TODAY

What I want you both to know

Week 40 — PREGNANCY *Journal*

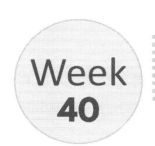

TOTAL WEIGHT GAIN

BELLY MEASUREMENT

BABY BUMP PHOTO

WEEKLY REFLECTIONS

SYMPTOMS & CRAVINGS

WHAT I WANT TO REMEMBER MOST

I'M MOST EXCITED ABOUT

I'M MOST NERVOUS ABOUT

Dear Babies,

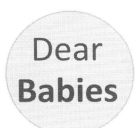

PREGNANCY *Journal*

TODAY'S DATE

WEEKS PREGNANT

HOW I'M FEELING TODAY

What I want you both to know

Made in the USA
Columbia, SC
09 February 2022